NOURISHING RECIPES FOR A DIVERTICULITIS-FRIENDLY LIFESTYLE

Delicious Recipes for Managing Irritable Bowel Syndrome and Diverticulitis Symptoms

Jasmine F. Lynch

TABLE OF CONTENTS

INTRODUCTION

Welcome to Delicious Healing: Nourishing Recipes for a Diverticulitis-Friendly Lifestyle! Living with diverticulitis can feel overwhelming as you try to balance maintaining a nutritious diet with managing painful symptoms. This cookbook was created to provide you with easy and delicious recipes that will help you to keep your diverticulitis under control. Each recipe is specifically tailored to help you adhere to a diverticulitis-friendly lifestyle, with nutrient-dense, gentle ingredients on the digestive system. This cookbook includes recipes for breakfast, lunch, dinner, snacks, desserts, and options for vegetarians and vegans. With these recipes, you'll be able to create simple and mouthwatering meals that can help to promote healing and ease the symptoms of diverticulitis. Get ready to nourish your body with Delicious Healing!

CHAPTER ONE: Understanding Diverticulitis: A Brief Overview

Diverticulitis is a condition that affects the large intestine, and if left untreated, can be very serious. It is caused by the inflammation of small pouches, known as diverticula, which form in the lining of the large intestine. In most cases, these pouches become infected, leading to a condition known as diverticulitis.

The main symptom of diverticulitis is abdominal pain, usually in the lower left side of the abdomen. Other symptoms include nausea, vomiting, chills, fever, and constipation. If the infection spreads, it can cause inflammation in other areas of the body, including the skin and bladder.

The exact cause of diverticulitis is unknown, but it's thought to be related to a poor diet lacking enough fiber. A lack of exercise can also contribute to this condition, as it can lead to constipation, which can put more pressure on the colon and irritate the diverticula.

The best way to treat diverticulitis is with diet and lifestyle changes. A diet rich in fiber helps to add bulk to stool so it moves more easily through the intestine. Plenty of fruit, vegetables, grains, and legumes are recommended for optimal digestive health. Additionally, exercising regularly and staying away from smoking can also help.

In more serious cases, antibiotics may be needed to treat the infection, and surgery may be advisable to remove the affected part of the intestine.

Embracing a Diverticulitis-Friendly Lifestyle

Diverticulitis can make life complicated, but thankfully there are ways to lead a healthier, more diverticulitis-friendly lifestyle. With thoughtful changes to your diet and an increase in exercise, you can work to reduce flare-ups and discomfort.

Foods to Limit

While a balanced diet is important for everyone, individuals with diverticulitis should be especially mindful of which foods they consume. Increased intake of refined grains and processed foods can be irritating to the digestive system and should be avoided. Additionally, foods high in saturated fat such as fried foods and red meat can be difficult to digest and tax the digestive system, so they should be limited.

Foods to Enjoy

On the other hand, a diet that is high in fiber can help reduce the risk of diverticulitis flare-ups. To meet your daily dietary fiber needs, opt for a variety of fruits, vegetables, legumes, and whole grains. These types of foods are easier to digest and can help you stay regular.

Exercise

Exercising regularly can also have positive effects on diverticulitis. Even low-intensity activities such as walking or swimming can help improve blood flow and reduce inflammation. Light strength training can also benefit you if your doctor or healthcare provider approves.

Lifestyle Adjustments

Finally, making lifestyle adjustments such as reducing stress, managing anxiety, and getting adequate sleep can also help manage diverticulitis flare-ups. Smoking and alcohol use should be avoided, as these substances can be detrimental to your overall digestive health.

With these tips, you can take steps to manage your diverticulitis and make the most of your life. The recipes in this cookbook will also help you find delicious, diverticulitis-friendly options to include in your mealtime routine. So, take proactive measures and embrace a healthier lifestyle for your digestive health!

CHAPTER TWO: Essential Nutrients and Ingredients

Key Nutrients for Digestive Health

The gastrointestinal tract is an essential component of overall health and nutrition, so it is important to be aware of what key nutrients are necessary to promote digestive health. Here are some key nutrients that play a role in digestive health.

1. Fiber

Fiber is important for digestive health because it absorbs water, which increases the bulk of the stool, aiding in its passage through the body. It also serves as a source of fuel for beneficial intestinal bacteria. Sources of fiber include fruits, vegetables, and whole grains.

2. Probiotics

Probiotics are beneficial bacteria that are essential for a healthy digestive system. They help to break down food, absorb nutrients, and protect against infections. Probiotics can be found in yogurt, kefir, kimchi, tempeh, and supplements.

3. Prebiotics

Prebiotics are indigestible carbohydrates and fiber that serve as fuel for the beneficial bacteria in the gut. Sources of prebiotics include bananas, garlic, onions, asparagus, oats, and legumes.

4. Omega-3 Fatty Acids

Omega-3 fatty acids are essential fatty acids that are important for digestive health, as they help to reduce inflammation and protect the lining of the gut. Sources of omega-3 fatty acids include fish, walnuts, flaxseeds, and canola oil.

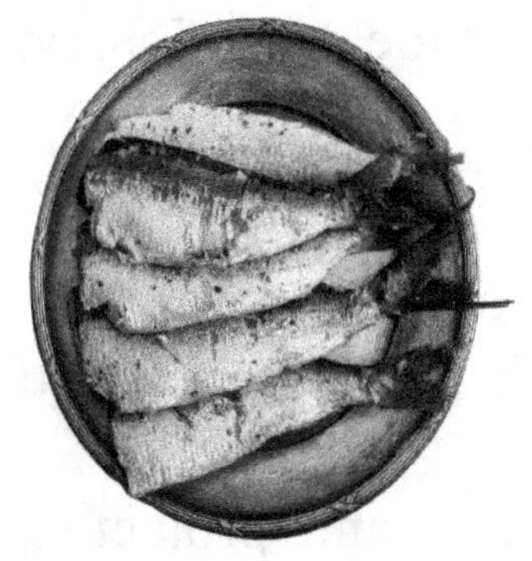

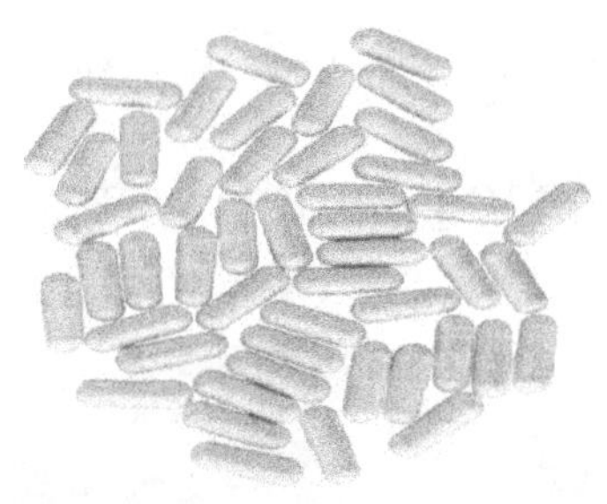

5. Protein

Protein is important for digestive health since it helps to repair and build the muscles in the lining of the gut. Additionally, it also helps to produce enzymes that aid in digestion.

Sources of protein include meat, fish, poultry, eggs, nuts, and legumes.

These key nutrients are necessary to support digestive health as they help to break down food, absorb nutrients, and protect against infections. Consuming a diet rich in these nutrients will ensure that your body is getting all the necessary nutrients to promote optimal digestive health.

Selecting the Right Ingredients: Fiber-Rich and Gut-Friendly Choices

Your gut health is connected to overall well-being, and selecting the right ingredients for your meals can play an important role in maintaining it. Eating more fiber-rich foods and choosing those that are more gut-friendly can help to regulate digestion and promote a healthy gut microbiome.

When selecting ingredients that are both fiber-rich and gut-friendly, the most important thing to consider is the type of fiber they contain. For optimal gut health, dietary fibers are best divided into two categories: insoluble fiber and soluble fiber.

Insoluble fiber is the type of fiber that is not broken down in the body and is especially beneficial for digestion. It helps add bulk to stools and can help alleviate constipation. Good sources of insoluble fiber include whole-grain bread and cereals, wheat bran, nuts and seeds, legumes, and potatoes.

Soluble fiber, on the other hand, is broken down in your body and is known to help lower cholesterol levels, stabilize blood sugar levels, and reduce the risk of heart disease. Good sources of soluble fiber include oatmeal, barley, beans, peas, apples, oranges, pears, flax seeds, and chia seeds.

When shopping for ingredients that are both fiber-rich and gut-friendly, it is important to look for those that are minimally processed and contain no added preservatives. Whole grains, fruits, vegetables, nuts, and seeds are all great options. If shopping for canned goods, be sure to check the ingredients list for added sugars, salt, and preservatives.

It can also be beneficial to include probiotic and fermented foods, such as yogurt, sauerkraut, and kimchi in your diet. These foods contain beneficial bacteria that can help balance the gut microbiome. Adding a few servings of these foods to your diet each week can provide numerous health benefits.

Finally, be sure to drink plenty of water throughout the day. Staying hydrated helps to regulate digestion and can also help keep your gut healthy.

By following these simple tips for selecting ingredients that are both fiber-rich and gut-friendly, you can incorporate the healthiest and most nourishing foods into your diet. This will help you fuel your body with the nutrients it needs daily and aid in promoting optimal gut health.

CHAPTER THREE: Breakfast Beginnings

Creamy Banana-Oat Smoothie

Creamy Banana-Oat Smoothies are the perfect drink to help maintain a healthy and nutritious diet. The smoothie is packed with color and flavor and provides a great way to start your day. Here's how to make a creamy banana-oat smoothie in just a few easy steps.

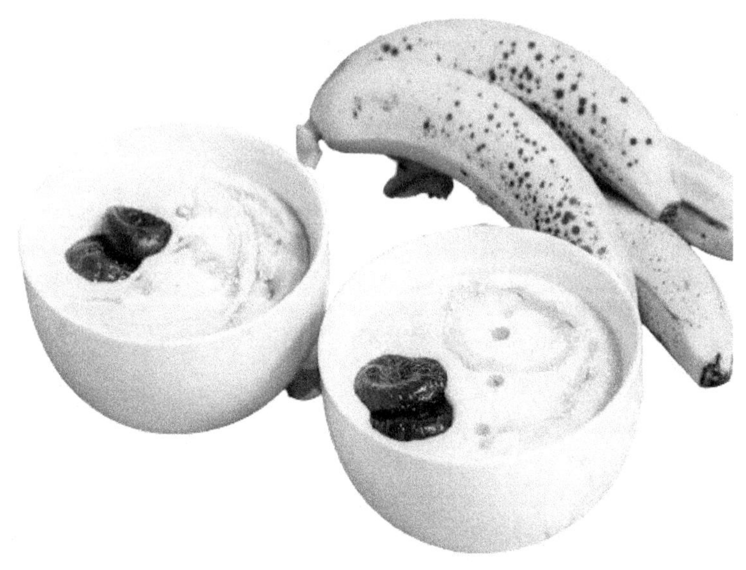

Ingredients:

- ½ cup rolled oats

- ½ cup plain yogurt

- 1 banana

- ½ cup almond milk

- ½ teaspoon of vanilla extract

- Honey to taste (optional)

1. Place rolled oats, yogurt, banana, almond milk, and vanilla extract in a blender and process until completely combined.

2. Pour the mixture into a glass.

3. Add a dash of honey for sweetness, if desired.

4. Garnish with fresh banana slices for a presentation.

And there you have it – an easy, healthy, and delicious creamy banana-oat smoothie that will help you start your day off with a nutritious breakfast.

Quinoa Breakfast Bowl with Berries

Add a healthy and delicious new spin to your breakfast with this delicious Quinoa Breakfast Bowl with Berries. This breakfast bowl is a great way to get in the essential nutrients and fiber that you need to make sure that you are following a good diverticulitis diet.

Ingredients:

-1 cup cooked quinoa

-1/2 cup fresh blueberries

-1/2 cup fresh blackberries

-1/4 cup raw almonds, chopped

-1 tablespoon honey

-1/4 teaspoon ground cinnamon

-1/4 teaspoon ground nutmeg

-2 tablespoons almond milk

-1 teaspoon lemon zest

Instructions:

1. In a medium bowl, combine the cooked quinoa, blueberries, blackberries, chopped almonds, honey, cinnamon, nutmeg, almond milk, and lemon zest. Stir until the ingredients are well combined.

2. Divide the quinoa mixture into two bowls.

3. Top each bowl with a few extra blueberries and blackberries.

4. Serve the breakfast bowls warm and enjoy!

Serving size	Calories	Fat (g)	Carbohydrates(g)	Fiber(g)	Protein(g)
1 bowl	347	9.6	53	8.1	10

This recipe is a great way to start the day on the right foot with a nutritious diverticulitis diet-friendly breakfast. Enjoy!

Flaxseed and Blueberry Muffins

As you're managing your diverticulitis symptoms, you don't have to abandon tasty foods that you enjoy. Flaxseed and blueberry muffins are a nutrient-rich snack with just the right amount of sweetness. Eating healthy snacks like these muffins can help you stay on track while still giving you a yummy treat.

These muffins are bursting with dietary fiber. They contain flaxseed, white whole wheat flour, and oat bran, which all contribute toward your daily fiber intake. Flaxseed also provides healthy omega-3 fatty acids, which are important for a good diet. For those of you looking to reduce your use of processed sugar, this recipe utilizes the natural sweetness of blueberries as an alternative.

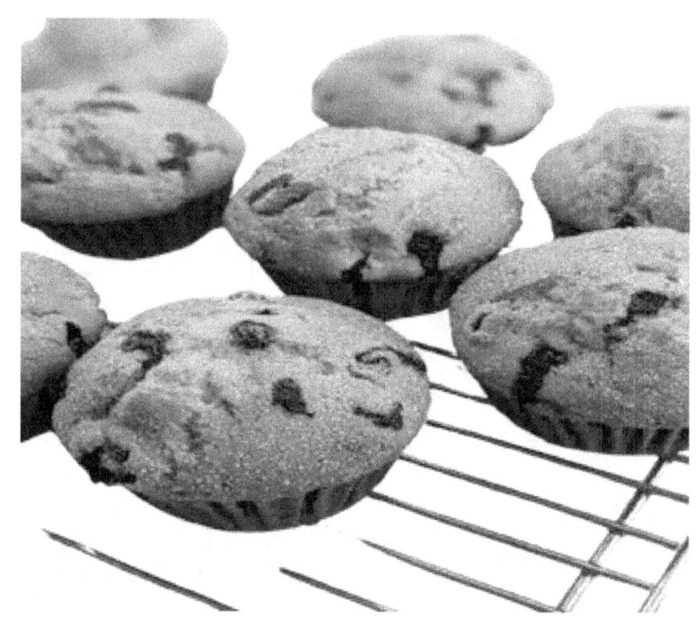

-1 cup white whole-wheat flour

-1/2 cup oat bran

-1/4 cup ground flaxseed

-1 teaspoon baking powder

-1 teaspoon baking soda

-1/4 teaspoon ground cinnamon

-1/4 teaspoon ground nutmeg

-1/2 teaspoon salt

-1/2 cup plain, non-dairy yogurt

-1/3 cup honey

-1/4 cup olive oil

-1 teaspoon vanilla extract

-1 cup fresh blueberries

First, preheat your oven to 400°F. Grease a muffin tin or a silicone muffin tin with olive oil. In a medium-sized bowl, mix the white whole wheat flour, oat bran, ground flaxseed, baking powder, baking soda, cinnamon, nutmeg, and salt.

In a separate large bowl, whisk together the yogurt, honey, olive oil, and vanilla extract. Slowly mix in the dry ingredients, then fold in the blueberries. Fill each muffin cup three-quarters of the way full and top with a sprinkle of oat bran, if desired.

Bake for 18-20 minutes or until a toothpick inserted in the center comes out clean. When the muffins have cooled enough to handle, store them in an airtight container for up to one week or freeze them if desired.

CHAPTER FOUR: Wholesome Soups and Nourishing Stews

Healing Chicken and Vegetable Broth

Diverticulitis can be a painful and uncomfortable condition, making it difficult to eat or enjoy many of your favorite foods. Luckily, one flavorful dish that is suitable for this condition is healing chicken and vegetable broth. Packed with nutritious vegetables, soothing herbs, and flavorful broth, it's an ideal meal for anyone suffering from diverticulitis.

In this chapter, we'll explore the benefits of chicken and vegetable broth for people suffering from diverticulitis, learn how to choose the right ingredients and make a simple and delicious healing broth. By the time you're finished, you'll be able to make a meal that's easy to digest and nourishing and will restore your gut health.

Benefits of Chicken and Vegetable Broth

Chicken and vegetable broth offers several benefits for those suffering from diverticulitis. It contains natural antioxidants, minerals, and vitamins that help reduce inflammation and restore gut health. This type of broth also provides an excellent source of protein, which helps build and maintain healthy muscles. Further, it's easy to digest and contains fiber, which helps to soften and move stools.

How to Choose Ingredients

To make a flavorful and nutritious chicken and vegetable broth, it's important to choose the right ingredients. Start with low-sodium chicken broth, as it eliminates the need to add extra salt and helps keep your sodium intake in check.

For vegetables, choose a variety of colors such as carrots, celery, onions, garlic, mushrooms, and leeks. These vegetables contain antioxidants and prebiotics, which help balance gut flora and aid in digestion.

Finally, include herbs such as thyme, oregano, parsley, and bay leaves. Not only do these herbs add flavor and aroma, but they also contain prebiotics and antioxidants that can also help reduce inflammation and improve gut health.

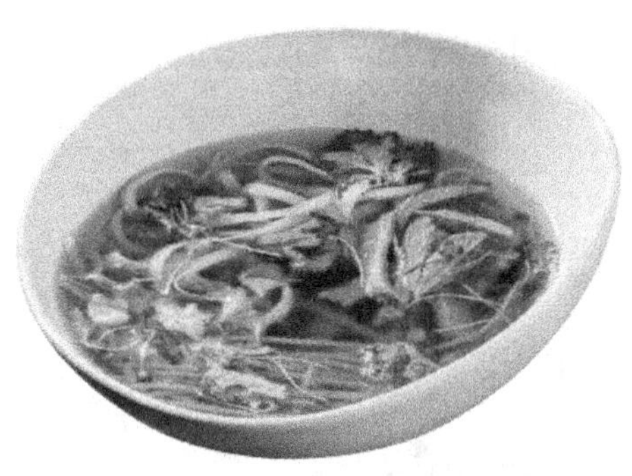

Ingredients:

-1-quart low-sodium chicken broth

-1 small onion, chopped

-1 large carrot, diced

-2 stalks of celery, diced

-2 cloves garlic, minced

-1 cup mushrooms, finely chopped

- Leek, thinly sliced

-1 tablespoon fresh thyme

-1 teaspoon dried oregano

-1 teaspoon dried parsley

-1 bay leaf

Instructions:

1. In a large pot, combine chicken broth, onion, carrot, celery, garlic, mushrooms, and leek.

2. Bring to a boil over high heat. Reduce heat to low and simmer for 20 minutes.

3 Add remaining ingredients and simmer for an additional 10 minutes.

4. Remove from heat and let cool slightly. Strain broth and serve.

Enjoy your healing chicken and vegetable broth to support your gut health and reduce inflammation. This mild broth is easy to digest and packed with nutrition to help you heal from diverticulitis.

Creamy Potato Leek Soup

Prep time: 10 minutes

Cook time: 25 minutes

Serves: 4

Potato leek soup is a classic comfort food dish that can easily be adapted for those with diverticulitis. This creamy version pairs potatoes with leeks, vegetable stock, and cream for a hearty and flavorful soup that is sure to satisfy.

Ingredients:

- 2 tablespoons butter

- 2 medium leeks, white and light green parts only, thinly sliced

- 4 small russet potatoes, peeled and diced

- 4 cups low-sodium vegetable stock

- 1 cup heavy cream

- Salt and freshly ground black pepper, to taste

<u>***Instructions:***</u>

1. In a large pot over medium-high heat, melt the butter. Add the leeks and sauté until softened, about 5 minutes.

2. Add the potatoes and stock to the pot. Bring to a boil, then reduce the heat to medium-low and simmer for 15 minutes or until the potatoes are tender.

3. Remove the pot from the heat and use an immersion blender to puree the soup until smooth.

4. Stir in the cream and season with salt and pepper to taste.

5. Divide the soup among four bowls and serve.

Lentil and Spinach Stew

Lentil and spinach stew is a hearty and nutritious meal that is full of flavorful, easy-to-digest ingredients. As part of a diverticulitis-friendly diet, this stew is low in insoluble fiber and high in soluble fiber, making it gentle on the digestive system. Lentils are a great source of protein and minerals, and spinach is packed with vitamins and minerals. This stew can be customized to your taste, adding vegetables and herbs for extra flavor.

Ingredients:

- 2 tablespoons extra-virgin olive oil

- 1 small onion, chopped

- 2 cloves garlic, minced

- 2 carrots, diced

- 1 celery stalk, diced

- 1 teaspoon dried oregano

- 2 cups low-sodium vegetable broth

- 1 cup dried lentils

- 1 bay leaf

- 2 cups fresh spinach leaves

- Salt and pepper, to taste

- Optional: Chopped fresh parsley, for garnish

Instructions:

1. Heat the oil in a large pot over medium-high heat. Add the onion, garlic, carrot, and

celery and cook until the vegetables are tender about 5 minutes.

2. Add the oregano, vegetable broth, lentils, and bay leaf. Simmer the stew until the lentils are tender, about 30 minutes.

3. Add the spinach and stir to combine. Simmer until the spinach is wilted, about 10 minutes.

4. Remove from heat and season to taste with salt and pepper. Divide into bowls and garnish with parsley, if desired.

Enjoy this delicious and nutritious stew on its own or with a side of cooked quinoa, couscous, or grits for a complete meal. This stew can be stored in the fridge for up to three days or can be frozen for up to three months.

Lentils and spinach make a great combination when cooked together for a hearty stew. The perfect combination of soluble and insoluble fiber makes this an ideal meal for those dealing with diverticulitis.

CHAPTER FIVE: Salads for Wellness

Grilled Salmon and Mixed Greens Salad

This fresh and flavorful dish is perfect for those suffering from diverticulitis! Grilled salmon provides the protein you need to keep your digestive tract healthy, while the bounty of greens gives you all the essential vitamins and minerals you need. This dish can be served as a main course, a starter, or a side dish, and can be served warm or cold.

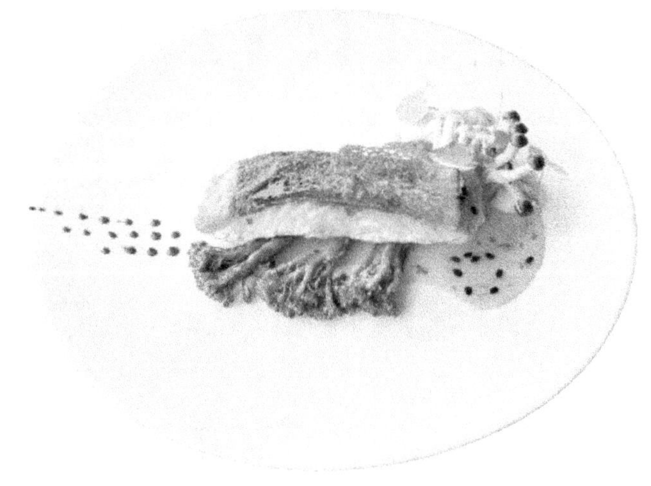

Ingredients:

- 4 salmon fillets

- 2 tablespoons olive oil

- 2 cloves garlic, minced

- 1 teaspoon of sea salt

- 1 teaspoon freshly ground black pepper

- 4 cups mixed greens

- 1/4 cup balsamic vinegar

- 2 tablespoons olive oil

- 1 teaspoon honey

- 1 tablespoon lemon juice

Instructions:

1. Heat a large non-stick skillet over high heat.

2. Brush two tablespoons of olive oil over the salmon fillets and season with garlic, sea salt, and black pepper.

3. Carefully place the fillets in the hot skillet and cook for 7-8 minutes, flipping once. When cooked through, remove from the heat and set aside.

4. In a large bowl, toss the mixed greens with balsamic vinegar, olive oil, honey, and lemon

juice. Taste and adjust the seasoning to your liking.

5. Place the salad onto plates and top with the cooked salmon fillets. Serve warm or cold.

Citrus Quinoa Salad with Avocado

Welcome to your delicious and nutritious Citrus Quinoa Salad with Avocado! This dish makes for a great side dish or light lunch. Eating a variety of foods is a great way to keep your gut healthy with diverticulitis. Quinoa is a great source of fiber and other nutrients and a mainstay in a diverticulitis diet. The citrus and avocado in this recipe add a bright zing of flavor and lots of beneficial vitamins and minerals.

To Make Citrus Quinoa Salad with Avocado:

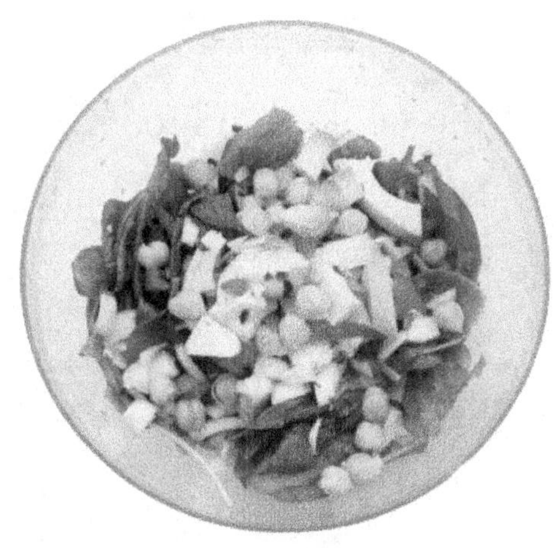

Ingredients:

-1 cup cooked quinoa

-1/2 of red onion, finely diced

-1 red bell pepper, diced

-1 avocado, diced

- Juice of 1 lime

- 1 tablespoon of extra virgin olive oil

- Salt and pepper to taste

Instructions:

1. Combine the cooked quinoa, diced onion, and diced red pepper in a medium mixing bowl.

2. In a separate small bowl, mix the lime juice and olive oil.

3. Pour the lime juice and olive oil mixture over the quinoa salad mixture and toss to combine.

4. Gently stir in the diced avocado.

5. Season with salt and pepper to taste and serve.

Enjoy!

This Citrus Quinoa Salad with Avocado is a great way to get a variety of heart-healthy ingredients into your diet. Quinoa is an excellent source of fiber and other nutrients, and with the addition of avocado and citrus, you'll get an added boost of vitamins and minerals. Enjoy this dish as a side with your favorite diverticulitis-friendly meals.

Roasted Vegetable Medley with Pesto Dressing

This Roasted Vegetable Medley with Pesto Dressing is a great, delicious, and nutritious dish that's ideal for those with Diverticulitis. Roasting vegetables tend to bring out their natural sweetness and nuttiness, making them a perfect bed for pesto, which can equally be flavorful, while not being too heavy on your belly. It's an easy-to-make dinner that's sure to please the palate of anyone with diverticulitis.

Ingredients:

-2 tablespoons olive oil

-1 red onion, chopped

-1 red pepper, chopped

-1 yellow pepper, chopped

-1 large corvette, chopped

-1 carrot peeled and chopped

-Salt and pepper to taste

-2 cloves garlic, minced

-2 tablespoons thinly sliced fresh basil

-4 tablespoons pesto

-1 tablespoon red wine vinegar

Instructions:

1. Preheat your oven to 200C.

2. In a medium bowl, combine the olive oil, chopped vegetables, salt and pepper. Mix them all together until the olive oil coats all of the vegetables.

3. Place the mixed vegetables onto a parchment-lined baking sheet. Ensure that the vegetables are spread out to ensure even roasting.

4. Roast the vegetables for 25 minutes, flipping them over halfway through. You will

want the vegetables to be lightly browned and caramelized.

5. In the meantime, mix the garlic, basil, pesto, and red wine vinegar to create the pesto dressing.

6. Once the vegetables have finished roasting, transfer them to a serving dish and top with the pesto dressing. Serve hot.

Enjoy this delicious roasted vegetable medley with pesto dressing as a side dish, or as the main event - either way, it's a flavorful and healthy dish that's made with foods that are easy to digest!

CHAPTER SIX:
Gut-Healing
Entrees

Baked Herb-Crusted Chicken

This flavorful Baked Herb-Crusted Chicken is perfect for a diverticulitis diet, as it is low in fat and rich in flavor. Not only is it nutritious and delicious, but it is also easy to prepare. This is a great weeknight meal that the whole family will enjoy.

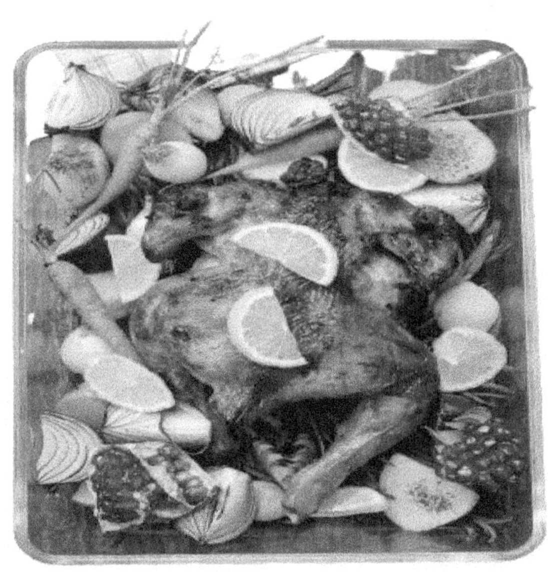

Ingredients

- 2 boneless, skinless chicken breasts

- ½ cup almond flour

- 2 tablespoons fresh oregano, finely chopped

- 2 tablespoons fresh parsley, finely chopped

- 2 tablespoons fresh thyme, finely chopped

- 2 tablespoons extra-virgin olive oil

- 1 teaspoon garlic powder

- ½ teaspoon onion powder

- ½ teaspoon sea salt

- ¼ teaspoon ground black pepper

Instructions

1. Preheat the oven to 400°F/204°C.

2. Place the chicken breasts in a baking dish.

3. In a small bowl, combine the almond flour, oregano, parsley, thyme, olive oil, garlic powder, onion powder, sea salt, and pepper. Stir until well combined.

4. Spread the herb mixture evenly over the chicken breasts, making sure to coat them completely.

5. Bake for 20 minutes, or until the chicken is cooked through.

6. Serve with your favorite sides and enjoy!

Healthy eating doesn't have to be boring!

Ginger-Glazed Carrot and Tempeh Stir-Fry

The Ginger-Glazed Carrot and Tempeh Stir-Fry is a tasty vegetarian meal that is full of fiber and nutrition. It is perfect for those following a diverticulitis-friendly diet as it is low in fat and contains complex carbohydrates. This stir-fry is also rich in beta-carotene, protein, calcium, magnesium, and iron, making it a great option for a healthy meal.

Ingredients:

- 2 tablespoons of canola oil

-1/2 teaspoon of freshly grated ginger

- 2 cloves of garlic, minced

- 1/2 cup of carrots, sliced

- 1/2 cup of tempeh, cubed

- 1/2 cup of snow peas, trimmed

- 1/4 cup of vegetable stock

- 2 tablespoons of soy sauce

- 2 tablespoons of honey

Instructions:

1. Heat the oil in a large skillet over medium heat.

2. Add the ginger and garlic and cook for 1-2 minutes, stirring occasionally.

3. Add the carrots, tempeh, and snow peas to the skillet and cook for 5 minutes, stirring occasionally.

4. Add the vegetable stock, soy sauce, and honey to the skillet and cook for an additional 5 minutes, stirring occasionally.

5. Turn off the heat and serve, garnishing with extra ginger if desired.

Enjoy this delicious and nutritious dish as part of a diverticulitis-friendly diet!

Serving size	1 bowl
Calories	229
Fat(g)	8.7
Carbs(g)	27.2
Fiber(g)	8.1
Protein(g)	14.4
S0dium (mg)	911

Seared Cod with Lemony Asparagus

Seared cod and lemony asparagus make a simple and delicious combination that is full of flavor and nutrition! This dish is also perfect for those with Diverticulitis, as it is low in fiber and contains healthy omega-3 fatty acids. Why not give it a try this week?

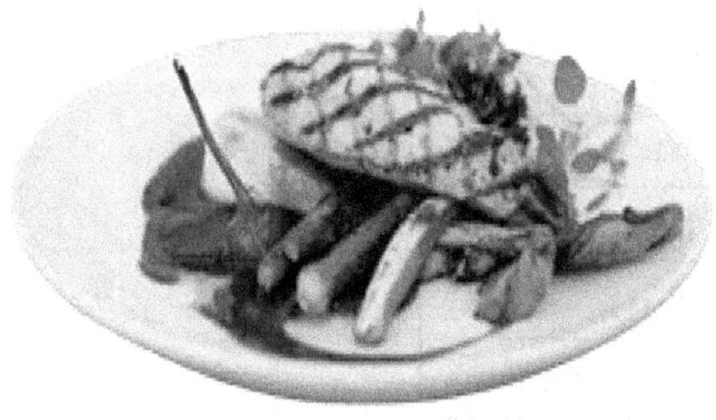

Ingredients:

- 4 Cod fillets

- 1 bunch of Asparagus

- 1 Lemon

- 2 tablespoons Olive Oil

- Salt and Pepper to taste

<u>*Instructions:*</u>

1. Preheat oven to 400 degrees.

2. Cut the asparagus into 2-inch pieces.

3. In a large bowl, combine the asparagus with olive oil and a pinch of salt and pepper.

4. Spread the asparagus onto a baking sheet and roast for about 15 minutes.

5. Meanwhile, season the cod fillets with salt and pepper.

6. Heat a skillet over medium-high heat and add a tablespoon of olive oil.

7. Carefully place the cod fillets in the pan and cook for about 3-4 minutes per side, until golden brown and cooked through.

8. Once the cod is cooked, remove from the heat and transfer to a plate.

9. Squeeze the juice of one lemon over the asparagus, toss gently, and serve alongside the cod.

Enjoy your Seared Cod with Lemony Asparagus! It makes for a quick and nutritious meal with minimal effort!

Give it a try and experience the joys of healthy home cooking. Bon Appétit!

CHAPTER SEVEN: Satisfying Sides and Snacks

Sweet Potato and Kale Hash

When it comes to eating for diverticulitis, incorporating fiber-rich and nutrient-packed vegetables such as sweet potatoes and kale is a surefire option. In this chapter, we'll be introducing you to a delicious recipe that you can add to your arsenal of diverticulitis-friendly meals—Sweet Potato and Kale Hash!

Ingredients

- 2 tablespoons olive oil

- 1 onion, diced

- 2 cloves garlic, minced

- 1 sweet potato, cubed

- 2 cups chopped kale

- Salt and pepper, to taste

- 2–3 tablespoons chopped fresh parsley

Instructions

1. Heat the oil in a large skillet over medium heat. Add the onion and garlic, and cook until the onion is softened and lightly golden, about 5 minutes.

2. Add the sweet potato cubes and cook until the potato starts to soften about 5 minutes.

3. Add the kale and season with salt and pepper. Cook, stirring often, until the kale has wilted and the sweet potato is cooked through about 5 minutes.

4. Serve the hash sprinkled with fresh parsley (if desired).

Enjoy!

Tips

• Not a fan of sweet potatoes? Feel free to substitute with any root vegetable of your choice.

• For extra flavor, you can also add a sprinkle of red pepper flakes, a few dashes of smoked paprika, or a small handful of crumbled feta cheese for richness.

• If you want to add a little protein to the mix, try topping the hash with poached, fried, or scrambled eggs.

• If you like your hash extra crispy, try baking it in the oven instead of cooking it on the stove. Just spread the prepared ingredients onto a baking sheet and bake at 400°F for 25–30 minutes.

Hummus and Veggie Platter

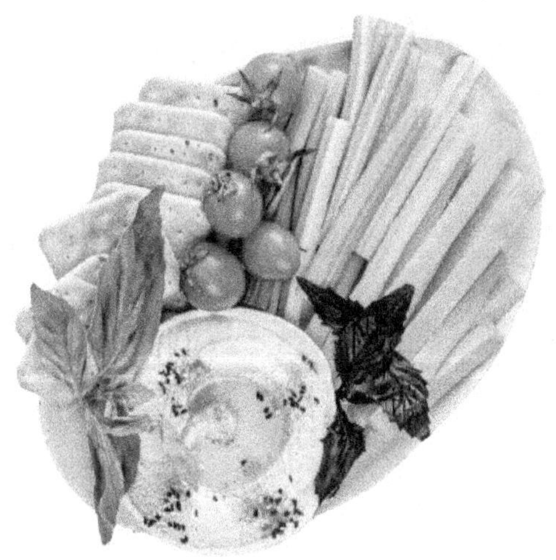

Hummus and veggie platters are a great way to get a healthy and nutritious meal that is easy to make and is especially beneficial for people on a diverticulitis diet. This dish is a great way to get your daily intake of vegetables without feeling like you are missing out on something due to dietary restrictions.

The base of the hummus and veggie platter should include a variety of crisp vegetables, such as raw carrots, celery, bell peppers, cucumbers, and cherry tomatoes. You can use store-bought hummus or make your own by blending cooked chickpeas with tahini, garlic, lemon juice, and a dash of olive oil. Spread the creamy hummus onto a plate or platter and arrange the vegetables around it.

Try adding different flavors and textures to your hummus and veggie platter. Nuts and seeds such as pumpkin or sesame are a great way to add a crunchy texture and additional flavor. Olives and artichokes provide a salty kick in addition to their rich nutrients. You can also add grilled peppers, or roasted sweet potatoes to your platter for extra flavor and nutrition.

If you are feeling adventurous, you can try adding vegan cheese and vegan meats that are commonly found in supermarkets. Just make sure that they are specifically designed to be vegan (e.g., no dairy, eggs, or fish products).

Serve your hummus and veggie platter with whole-grain pitas, or crackers for dipping.

Add a side of olives, hummus, and pickled vegetables for a full meal. Enjoy your hummus and veggie platter knowing that you are getting healthy and nutritious food in your diet.

Zucchini Fritters with Greek Yogurt Dip

Zucchini fritters are a great way to get more vegetables into your diet. The Greek yogurt dip is a delightful accompaniment to the fritters and helps add flavor and creaminess to the dish. The combination of both elements makes for a nutritious and delicious snack or light meal which is sure to be a hit with all the family.

Ingredients   (for   the fritters):

-2 medium zucchini, grated

-1/4 cup chives, diced

-1/4 cup basil, diced

-1/4 cup flat-leaf parsley, finely chopped

-1/4 cup parmesan cheese, grated

-2 cloves garlic, crushed

-1/2 cup Panko breadcrumbs

-1 egg

-Salt and pepper, to taste

-3 tablespoons olive oil

Ingredients (for the Greek yogurt dip):

-1/2 cup Greek yogurt

-1/4 cup lemon juice

-1/4 cup flat-leaf parsley, finely chopped

-1/2 teaspoon garlic powder

-1/2 teaspoon crushed red pepper flakes

-Salt and pepper, to taste

Instructions:

1. In a medium bowl, combine the grated zucchini, herbs, parmesan cheese, garlic, Panko breadcrumbs, egg, salt, and pepper.

2. Form the mixture into small patties and place them on a plate.

3. Heat the olive oil in a large non-stick skillet over medium heat.

4. Carefully place the fritters in the skillet and cook for about 2 minutes on each side, until golden brown.

5. To make the dip, combine the Greek yogurt, lemon juice, chopped parsley, garlic powder, red pepper flakes, salt, and pepper in a small bowl.

6. Serve the fritters with the dip and enjoy!

These zucchini fritters are a great addition to the diverticulitis diet as they are low in fat and contain lots of beneficial vegetables. Serve them as a delicious snack or light meal for the whole family and enjoy the health benefits of zucchini.

CHAPTER EIGHT: Comforting Casseroles and Bakes

Spinach and Ricotta Stuffed Shells

Is there anything more satisfying than al dente pasta filled with a creamy, cheesy filling? If you have diverticular disease, the answer to that question is yes! Spinach and Ricotta Stuffed Shells are a delicious dish for those with diverticular disease, combining the creamy, cheesy flavors of ricotta with the nutritional benefits of spinach. These shells are a hearty meal in one, and are sure to be a hit with all your family and friends!

Ingredients:

- 1 package of jumbo shell pasta

- 2 tablespoons olive oil

- 1 onion, finely diced

- 2 cloves garlic, minced

- 2 cups ricotta cheese

- 2 cups spinach, chopped

- 1 cup grated Parmesan cheese

- 2 tablespoons fresh basil, chopped

- Salt and pepper, to taste

- 2 cups Marinara sauce

<u>*Instructions*</u>

1. Preheat oven to 350 degrees. Grease a 9x13 baking dish.

2. Cook the shell pasta in a large pot of salted boiling water until al dente, about 8 minutes. Drain well.

3. Heat the olive oil in a large skillet over medium heat. Add the onions and cook, stirring occasionally, until softened about 5 minutes. Add the garlic and cook for a few minutes more.

4. Add the ricotta, spinach, Parmesan, basil, salt, and pepper. Cook, stirring, until heated through. Remove from heat.

5. Spoon about 2 tablespoons of the ricotta mixture into each jumbo shell. Place the shells in the prepared baking dish.

6. Spoon the Marinara sauce over the shells.

7. Bake for 20 minutes, until the shells are heated through and the sauce is bubbling. Serve hot.

This dish is a tasty way to enjoy a traditional Italian meal and get some of your recommended fiber intake from spinach. Enjoy this vegetarian dish as a delicious side dish or the main meal. Bon Appetit!

Turkey and Quinoa Stuffed Bell Peppers

Turkey and Quinoa Stuffed Bell Peppers: A Savory Dish for the Diverticulitis Diet

Bell peppers, a member of the nightshade family and a cousin of the potato, are an abundant antioxidant-rich food that is ideal for those on a diet for diverticulitis management. Their bright colors add vibrancy to the plate, and their red, orange, and yellow hues add nutrient diversity. In this chapter of your healing-focused cookbook, you will create a savory dish for diverticulitis that combines the nutritional benefits of bell peppers with the high-protein of lean turkey and the fiber-rich quinoa for a complete meal.

Ingredients:

- 1 lb ground turkey

- 1 cup cooked quinoa

- 1/2 onion, finely diced

- 1/2 teaspoon oregano

- 1/4 teaspoon garlic powder

- 1/4 teaspoon paprika

- 1/4 teaspoon black pepper

- 4 bell peppers, tops removed and seeded

- 2 tablespoons extra-virgin olive oil

- 1/4 teaspoon salt

Instruction:

1. Preheat your oven to 375F.

2. In a large bowl, mix the ground turkey, cooked quinoa, onions, oregano, garlic powder, paprika, and black pepper.

3. Take the bell peppers and stuff with the turkey and quinoa mixture, pack tightly, and place into a greased baking dish.

4. Drizzle olive oil over the bell peppers and sprinkle salt.

5. Bake for 45 minutes until the bell peppers are tender and the turkey is cooked through.

6. Allow to cool before serving and enjoy.

When the bell peppers are eaten, the sweet-tart flavor of the pepper blends with the flavor-filled turkey and quinoa to create a dish that is both pleasing to the palate and beneficial for those with diverticulitis.

The turkey provides the lean protein that can help power through the day while the quinoa is an excellent source of Omega-3 fatty acids, calcium, and magnesium, which help reduce inflammation that is associated with diverticulitis.

The bell peppers, which provide the bulk of the dish's nutrition, contain abundant amounts of carotenoids, which assist the immune system and soothe the lining of the stomach. When combined, these ingredients form a complete dish that can be enjoyed by those on a diverticulitis management diet.

Butternut Squash and Sage Lasagna

This Butternut Squash and Sage Lasagna is an amazing option for those with diverticulitis. Lasagna is a high-fiber pasta dish that is full of vegetables and provides a nutrient-rich meal. The combination of butternut squash and sage gives this dish a unique flavor that is sure to please any palate.

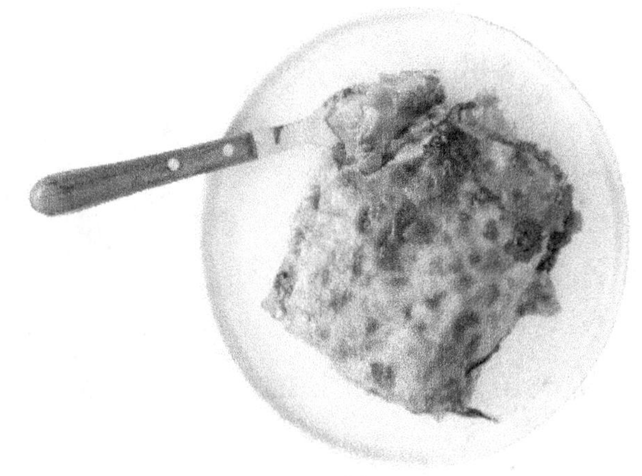

Ingredients:

-1 package of lasagna noodles

-2 tablespoons of olive oil

-1 small butternut squash peeled and cubed

-3 cloves of garlic, minced

-1 onion, diced

-2 cups of low-sodium chicken broth

-1 teaspoon of sugar

-1 teaspoon of dried sage

-Salt and pepper to taste

-2 cups of ricotta cheese

-1/2 cup of freshly grated Parmesan cheese

-1 cup of shredded mozzarella cheese

Instructions

1. Preheat oven to 375°F.

2. Bring a large pot of salted water to a boil. Add the lasagna noodles and cook until al dente. Drain and set aside.

3. Heat the olive oil in a large skillet over medium heat. Add the squash cubes, garlic,

and onion, and cook until the vegetables are tender.

4. Add the chicken broth, sugar, and sage, and season with salt and pepper. Simmer over low heat for 10 minutes until the liquid is thickened.

5. In a medium bowl, combine the ricotta, Parmesan, and mozzarella cheese.

6. To assemble the lasagna, spread a layer of the squash mixture in the bottom of a baking dish. Place a single layer of lasagna noodles on top. Spread a layer of cheese mixture over the noodles. Repeat the layering process with the remaining ingredients, ending with a layer of cheese.

7. Bake lasagna for 25-30 minutes, or until the cheese is golden and bubbly. Allow to cool for 10 minutes before serving. Enjoy!

CHAPTER NINE: Divine Desserts with a Twist

Berry Chia Seed Parfait

A Berry Chia Seed Parfait is a delicious and healthy option for someone with diverticulitis. This dish is packed with plenty of fiber-rich fruits and seeds that can help manage this condition and provide essential vitamins and minerals. With minimal prep time and easy ingredients, this parfait is a perfect choice for a quick and nutritious breakfast or snack.

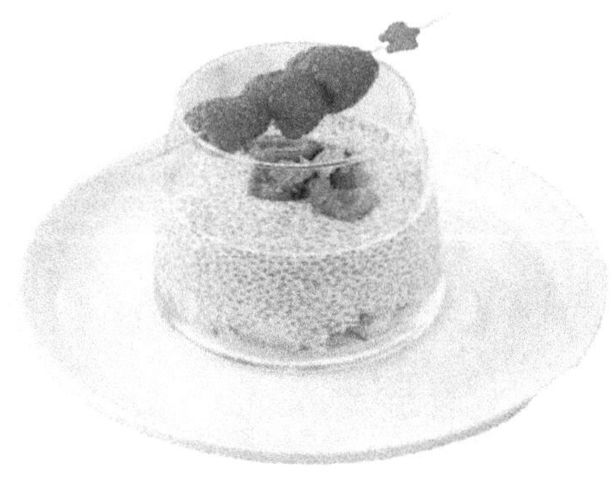

Ingredients:

-1/2 cup of dried fruit, such as dried cranberries or dried blueberries

-1 cup of your favorite fresh berries, such as blueberries, strawberries, or raspberries

-1/4 cup chia seeds

-1/4 cup of plain Greek yogurt

-1/4 cup of low-fat or non-fat milk

-1/4 cup of honey or agave

-1/2 teaspoon of ground cinnamon

-Optional: shredded coconut or granola for topping

Instructions:

1. Place the dried fruit in a small bowl and set aside.

2. In a separate bowl, combine the chia seeds, yogurt, milk, honey or agave, and cinnamon until fully incorporated. Let sit for 10 minutes to allow the chia seeds to absorb liquid and become gel-like.

3. In a large bowl, combine the fresh berries with the reserved dried fruit.

4. Take a small bowl, and spoon the chia seed mixture onto the bottom. Top with some of the berry and fruit mixture.

5. Layer again, repeating the process until all of the fruit has been used. For even layers, spoon the berry and fruit mixture in between each layer of the chia seed mixture.

6. Top with shredded coconut or granola, if desired.

7. Serve immediately or refrigerate for up to 3 days.

This Berry Chia Seed Parfait is a nutritious and delicious way to start the day for those suffering from diverticulitis. Not only does it provide loads of vitamins, minerals, and fiber, but it also has a great flavor and texture.

It can also be eaten as a snack throughout the day, providing a healthy and filling snack to tide you over until your next meal.

Baked Apples with Cinnamon and Walnuts

Are you ready for an easy and nutritious way to enjoy the flavor of apples with walnuts and cinnamon? If you are living with diverticulitis, this recipe is not only delicious, but it may also help reduce your symptoms.

This dish is a great way to add some required fiber to your diet. While fiber is not digested, insoluble fiber, which is found in nuts, apples, and wheat cereal, helps to soften stool and reduce pressure on the intestines. The soluble fiber found in oatmeal, applesauce, and dried peas can help reduce pain and diarrhea caused by diverticulitis.

Ingredients:

- 4 large apples

- ½ cup walnuts

- 2 tablespoons brown sugar

- 1 teaspoon ground cinnamon

- 2 tablespoons butter, melted

- ½ cup apple juice

Instructions:

1. Preheat oven to 350 degrees.

2. Core and slice apples; place in an 8x8 baking dish.

3. Sprinkle walnuts, brown sugar, and cinnamon over the apples.

4. Drizzle melted butter and apple juice over the top.

5. Bake in preheated oven for 30 minutes.

6. Serve warm.

This dish is a simple and delicious way to add additional fiber to your diet. It also provides a burst of flavor and nutrition.

Chocolate Avocado Mousse

Welcome to the world of healthy chocolate desserts! Of all the delicious, healthy desserts available to us these days, Chocolate Avocado Mousse stands out as one of the best. Rich and creamy, this recipe is perfect

for those with diverticulitis, as it is both tasty
and low in fiber.

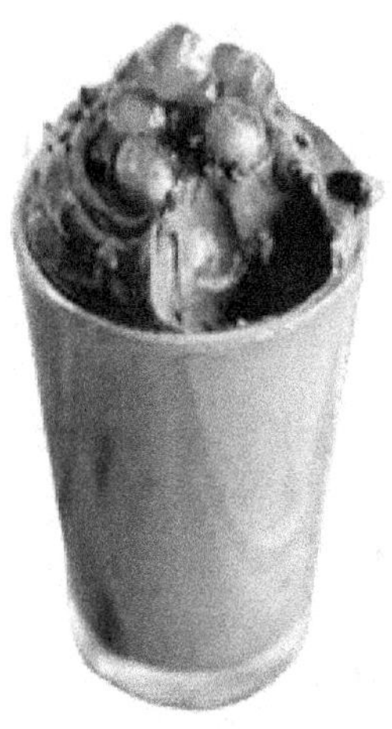

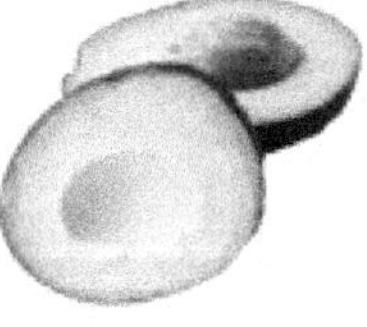

Ingredients

- 2 large ripe avocados

- ½ cup cocoa powder

- ¼ cup maple syrup

- 1 teaspoon vanilla extract

- ½ teaspoon salt

- ½ cup of coconut milk

Instruction

1. Cut the avocados in half, remove the pit, and scoop out the flesh using a spoon.

2. Place the avocado into a food processor, and add the cocoa, maple syrup, vanilla, and salt. Blend until creamy.

3. Add the coconut milk and continue to blend until the mousse is light and fluffy.

4. Refrigerate for at least an hour before serving.

As you have seen, making Chocolate Avocado Mousse is incredibly easy and takes very little time. Perfect for those with diverticulitis, this mousse is rich and creamy and won't aggravate your condition.

CHAPTER TEN: Drinks for Digestive Harmony

Fresh Ginger and Turmeric Infusion

Ginger and turmeric have long been used as traditional remedies for a variety of conditions. Studies have found that these herbs contain powerful anti-inflammatory properties that work to reduce inflammation in the digestive tract and help to reduce the symptoms of diverticulitis. In addition, ginger and turmeric provide powerful antioxidants that can help improve the immune system.

In this chapter, we will discuss the benefits of fresh ginger and turmeric, and how to create a simple infusion using these two herbs. This infusion will provide a refreshing alternative to traditional diverticulitis remedies and can be enjoyed as part of a delicious and nutritious diverticulitis diet.

Benefits of Ginger and Turmeric

Ginger and turmeric both have strong anti-inflammatory properties that can help to reduce inflammation in the digestive tract. These herbs also contain powerful antioxidants that can help to strengthen the immune system and prevent further disease.

Ginger is known to reduce nausea and improve digestion. It is great for reducing constipation, which is a common symptom of diverticulitis. Turmeric can help to reduce inflammation, reduce pain, and protect the digestive system.

How to Prepare a Fresh Ginger and Turmeric Infusion

To make a fresh ginger and turmeric infusion, you will need:

- 2 teaspoons of freshly grated ginger

- 2 teaspoons of freshly grated turmeric

- 2 cups of boiling water

Instructions:

1. Place the ginger and turmeric in a mug with boiling water.

2. Let the infusion steep for 10 minutes.

3. Strain the infusion into a clean mug.

4. Enjoy your infusion hot or cold.

Ginger and turmeric infusions are a delicious and refreshing way to add the healing benefits of these herbs to your diverticulitis diet. This simple infusion can also be a great substitute for coffee or tea. You can enjoy your ginger and turmeric infusion as part of a diverticulitis diet to support your digestive system and reduce the symptoms of diverticulitis.

Minty Cucumber-Lemon Water

Life on a diverticulitis diet doesn't have to be dull and uneventful. When hunger strikes, try quenching your thirst with this delicious and refreshing Minty Cucumber-Lemon Water. There are several benefits to drinking cucumber-lemon water that are especially helpful on a diverticulitis diet. Cucumbers and lemons are both sources of fiber, which is an essential part of a diverticulitis diet. Lemon juice helps to reduce inflammation, and its antioxidant properties help to boost your immune system. Mint adds a refreshing flavor to the drink and it can help to reduce inflammation and aid digestion.

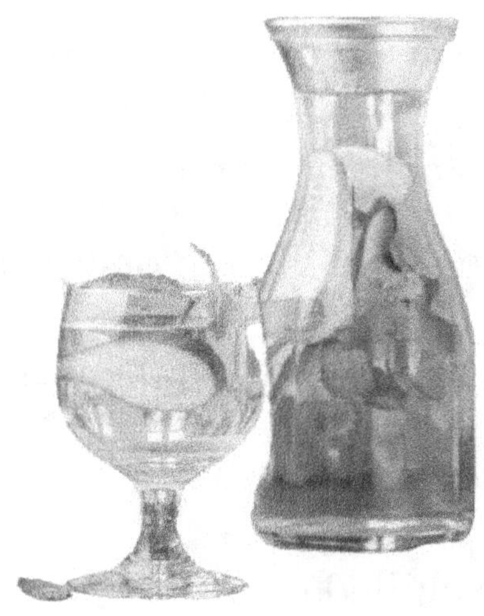

Ingredients:

- 2 cucumbers, thinly sliced

- 1 small lemon, thinly sliced

- 1/2 cup fresh mint leaves

- 2 quarts of filtered water

Directions:

1. In a large pitcher, combine the cucumbers, lemon slices, mint leaves, and water.

2. Stir to combine and let the mixture sit for 1 hour to allow the flavors to combine.

3. Strain the mixture into a pitcher or jar and discard the pulp.

4. Serve chilled or over ice.

Enjoy this refreshing and cooling Minty Cucumber-Lemon Water on a hot summer day, or any time! This delicious drink makes a great alternative to sugary juices or sodas while following a diverticulitis diet.

Herbal Teas for Soothing

Herbal teas can be a great way to soothe an inflamed intestine, help with digestion, and give comfort to those taking the diverticulitis diet. From ginger to peppermint, these teas can help calm and reduce inflammation in the digestive tract and reduce the incidence of flare-ups.

Ginger

Ginger is a popular herb that has long been used to calm the digestive system and reduce inflammation. It is widely used to treat gastrointestinal issues, including those related to diverticulitis. To make ginger tea, simply steep a teaspoon of freshly grated ginger in hot water for five minutes.

Chamomile

Chamomile has also been used for centuries to ease digestive upset and reduce inflammation and is widely used for the relief of diverticulitis. Making chamomile tea is simple. Steep a teaspoon of dried chamomile flowers in hot water for five minutes. Drink up to two times a day for best results.

Peppermint

Peppermint is another herb used to soothe the digestive system and calm an irritated intestine. Studies have shown that peppermint helps to reduce inflammation, as well as providing a sense of comfort. To make peppermint tea, steep a teaspoon of dried peppermint leaves in hot water for five minutes. You can drink up to three cups of this tea a day to soothe your diverticulitis.

Licorice

Licorice root has been used for centuries to help with a variety of digestive disorders, including diverticulitis. This herb helps to reduce inflammation and strengthens the protective lining of the stomach. To make licorice tea, steep a teaspoon of licorice root in hot water for five minutes. Limit your consumption of this tea to no more than two cups per day.

With these helpful herbal teas, you can soothe your digestive system and reduce the severity of your flare-ups related to diverticulitis. Adding these teas to your diet can be a gentle, natural way to help ease your pain and discomfort.

CHAPTER ELEVEN: Meal Planning and Preparation

For many people, diverticulitis is an uncomfortable gastrointestinal condition that can make meal planning and grocery shopping difficult. This chapter will provide weekly meal plans to help people find relief through on-trend strategies that promote diverticulitis wellness.

There are a few important considerations when following a diverticulitis-friendly diet. High-fiber foods can be hard to digest and can be painful for people with inflamed or irritated diverticula, so it is important to limit them. Whole grains should be replaced with refined grains, such as white rice or white flour, which are easier to digest. Additionally, increasing water intake can help promote digestive health. Lastly, it is important to take probiotics to help support the bacteria in the gastrointestinal tract and promote healthy digestion.

Weekly Meal Plans for Diverticulitis Wellness

A well-structured weekly meal plan can be a game-changer when it comes to managing diverticulitis and promoting digestive wellness. Here, you will find a comprehensive guide to creating balanced, flavorful, and nourishing meal plans that support your journey toward better health. Each meal plan is carefully crafted to incorporate a variety of nutrient-rich ingredients while taking into account the specific dietary needs of individuals with diverticulitis.

With that in mind, here is a sample plan for one week of meals that is compatible with a diverticulitis-friendly diet.

Sample Weekly Meal Plans:**

Note: These meal plans are provided as examples and can be adjusted based on your personal preferences and dietary requirements.

Monday

Breakfast: Scrambled eggs with mushrooms and bell peppers

Lunch: Grilled Salmon with mashed cauliflower

Dinner: Stuffed bell peppers

Tuesday

Breakfast: Greek Yogurt Parfait with Mixed Berries and Chia Seeds

Lunch: Tuna salad lettuce wrap

Dinner: Roasted turkey breast and steamed vegetables

Wednesday

Breakfast: Avocado toast

Lunch: Broiled salmon with quinoa

Dinner: Shrimp stir-fry with white rice

Thursday

Breakfast: Oats porridge with nuts and seeds

Lunch: Grilled chicken salad wrap

Dinner: Baked white fish with asparagus

Friday

Breakfast: Greek yogurt smoothie

Lunch: Lentil and Vegetable Soup with Whole Grain Roll

Dinner: Baked sweet potato with grilled vegetables

Saturday

Breakfast: Creamy Banana-Oat Smoothie

Lunch: Tuna salad sandwich

Dinner: Quinoa-Stuffed Bell Peppers with Side Salad

Sunday

Breakfast: Oatmeal pancake

Lunch: Grilled chicken wrap

Dinner: Baked cod with steamed broccoli.

Benefits of Weekly Meal Planning for Diverticulitis:

1. Consistency in Nutrition: Planning your meals ahead of time ensures that you consistently provide your body with the essential nutrients it needs to thrive, reducing the risk of flare-ups and discomfort.

2. Fiber Management: Strategic meal planning helps you incorporate the right amount of fiber into your diet without overwhelming your digestive system, promoting regular bowel movements and overall gut health.

3. Reduced Stress: With a meal plan in place, you can eliminate the daily stress of deciding what to eat, making grocery shopping more efficient, and minimizing the temptation to reach for less healthy options.

4. Controlled Portion Sizes: Portion control is crucial for diverticulitis management. By planning your meals, you can ensure that you're eating appropriate serving sizes and avoiding overeating.

Creating a Balanced Diverticulitis-Friendly Meal Plan:

When crafting your weekly meal plan, consider the following guidelines to ensure a well-balanced and nourishing approach:

1. Incorporate High-Fiber Foods: Choose a variety of fruits, vegetables, whole grains, legumes, and nuts that are rich in soluble and insoluble fiber. Gradually increase fiber intake to allow your digestive system to adjust.

2. Hydration: Include plenty of fluids, such as water, herbal teas, and infused waters, to help maintain proper hydration and support digestion.

3. Lean Proteins: Include lean sources of protein, such as poultry, fish, tofu, tempeh, and legumes, to support tissue repair and overall health.

4. Healthy Fats: Opt for heart-healthy fats from sources like avocados, nuts, seeds, and olive oil to promote satiety and provide essential nutrients.

5. Digestive Supplements: If advised by your healthcare provider, incorporate probiotics, prebiotics, and digestive enzymes into your meal plan to enhance gut health.

Tips for Preparing Diverticulitis-Friendly Meals

When it comes to preparing meals on the diverticulitis diet, you'll need to keep a few important points in mind. By following these tips, you'll be able to create a variety of meals that are both healthy and flavorful while also providing your body with the nutrients it needs to heal.

1. Choose Low-Fiber Foods: When choosing foods to include in your meals, be sure to prioritize those with a low-fiber content. High-fiber foods can be harder to digest and irritate the inflamed tissue in the intestine, making diverticulitis symptoms worse. Low-fiber foods that are great for a diverticulitis-friendly meal include white rice, white potatoes (without skin), peeled apples, bananas, cooked carrots, and yogurt.

2. Avoid Everyday Foods to Avoid: Certain everyday foods can aggravate diverticulitis symptoms, including popcorn, nuts, seeds, and corn. These hard-to-digest foods can get stuck in the ulcers in the intestine, so it's best to avoid them to avoid pain or discomfort.

3. Make It Easy to Digest: Certain cooking methods can make foods easier to digest. For example, opt for steamed or boiled vegetables rather than those that are fried. You should also opt for lean cuts of meat that have been cooked thoroughly to avoid any bacteria or parasites that could otherwise make the diverticulitis worse.

4. Vary Your Plate: As much as possible, you should try to include different types of low-fiber foods in your meals. Having a variety of flavors and textures on your plate can make the meal taste better and make it more likely that you'll get the nutrients you need.

5. Add Flavor: Low-fiber dishes can sometimes be bland, but that doesn't mean flavor should be sacrificed. Feel free to add extra seasonings, herbs, and spices to give the meal extra flavor. In addition to giving the food more flavor, some herbs and spices can also have certain health benefits for those with diverticulitis.

By following these tips, you can whip up delicious, diverticulitis-friendly meals that

both satisfy your cravings and help your body
heal.

CHAPTER TWELVE: Resources and Tips for Success

Shopping Guide: Stocking Your Diverticulitis Pantry

One of the major components of a healthy diet for someone suffering from diverticulitis is stocking the right type of food in the pantry. An effective way to manage your diverticulitis is to have a list of foods that are safe for you to eat on hand and a plan on how and when to eat them. That's why, in this chapter, we'll be going through the list of items you should have in your pantry.

Fiber

Fiber is important to any diet, but it is especially important for those with diverticulitis. When stocking up on fiber-rich foods, look for whole grains, nuts, fruits, and vegetables. Whole-wheat pasta, oats, nuts, and seeds are all excellent sources of fiber, as are high-fiber vegetables such as broccoli, spinach, and peas.

Starchy Vegetables

Starchy vegetables are rich in nutrients and low in calories, making them great for diverticulitis. Sweet potatoes and potatoes are excellent sources of fiber and complex carbohydrates as are corn, peas, and legumes.

Fruits

Fruits are a great source of vitamins, minerals, and fiber, which makes them a great part of the diverticulitis diet. Look for fresh or frozen fruits such as strawberries, blueberries, apples, oranges, bananas, kiwis, and mangos. Additionally, limit your intake of citrus fruits as they contain acids that may irritate the diverticula.

Proteins

Proteins are an essential part of the diverticulitis diet. Lean sources of proteins such as fish, poultry, and eggs are excellent sources of omega-3 fatty acids which can help reduce inflammation in the intestines. Beans and legumes are also excellent sources of proteins and can help provide additional fiber to the diet.

Healthy Fats

Healthy fats such as olive oil and avocados are essential to any diet. They help provide a healthy balance of essential nutrients and can help reduce inflammation. Additionally, look for sources of natural fats like nuts, seeds, coconut oil, and nut butter which make a great addition to any meal.

Herbs & Spices

When it comes to the diverticulitis diet, herbs and spices can be quite beneficial. Not only do they add flavor to meals, but they can also help reduce inflammation in the body. Look for dried and fresh herbs like oregano, basil, cumin, parsley, turmeric, ginger, and cinnamon. Additionally, look for fresh and dried spices like chili powder, cayenne, curry powder, and paprika, all of which can be a great addition to many recipes.

By stocking your pantry with these key ingredients, you'll be sure to have the necessary items to make tasty and nutritious meals. Follow this guide to ensure you have the right ingredients to maintain a balanced diverticulitis diet.

Dairy

Dairy can provide essential vitamins, minerals, and protein in the diverticulitis diet.

Choose low-fat varieties such as yogurt, low-fat milk, and cheese. Additionally, look for lactose-free options such as almond milk and lactose-free yogurt.

Other Staples

Other important items to have on hand in your diverticulitis pantry are broth, canned soups, peanut butter, honey, jams, and nut butter. Butter and margarine are other acceptable options but should be eaten in moderation. You can also include nuts on the diverticulitis diet but should avoid hard-to-digest varieties like peanuts and walnuts.

Managing Triggers and Flare-Ups

Diverticulitis is most commonly triggered by changes in the normal consistency of the stool. Changes in consistency can occur due to things such as stress, a change in diet, medication use, and even changes in the gut microbiome. Most people with diverticulitis notice certain foods to be a common trigger including foods high in fiber, high-fat foods, and carbonated beverages. It is important to note that everyone responds differently to food triggers and it may take some trial and error to figure out which foods cause flare-ups for you. Additionally, it is important to note that flares are not limited to food triggers. Other potential triggers can include disruption of your normal sleep cycle, extended periods of inactivity, episodes of stress, or other illnesses or medical conditions.

Once you are aware of what foods and situations are triggering diverticulitis flares and pain, there are management strategies to help minimize their effect. First, you should focus on following the diverticulitis diet including eating well-balanced meals, eating fiber-rich foods, limiting high-fat foods, and avoiding caffeine, alcohol, and carbonated beverages. Additionally, you should focus on managing stress and sleep patterns by incorporating regular exercise, relaxation techniques, and proper rest. If medications are prescribed to control pain, be sure to take them as directed.

Managing triggers and flare-ups of diverticulitis is key to reducing symptoms and improving overall health and well-being. By understanding the potential triggers, developing an individualized nutrition plan, and focusing on stress and sleep management, you can effectively manage diverticulitis flare-ups.

Finally, it is important to understand that flares and triggers will vary from person to person. Keeping a food diary or journal to track your meals, snacks, and flare-up symptoms may be helpful in better understanding your triggers and strategies will also help to prevent flare-ups.

Dining Out with Diverticulitis: Smart Choices

Even if you are on a diverticulitis diet, there is still no need to stay isolated from the dining-out experience. With the right knowledge and preparation, socializing with friends and family over meals while also following the diverticulitis diet is possible.

When making a restaurant reservation, let the waiter or waitress know that you require a diverticulitis-friendly meal. If the restaurant has an online menu, take a few minutes to check out their selection before dining out. Look for options that are low in fat, refined carbohydrates, and red meat, as these will be harder to digest and can cause a flare-up of symptoms. Also, be sure to ask about any hidden ingredients in prepared dishes such as sauces and gravies.

When ordering, focus on dishes that contain high-fiber, plant-based ingredients such as vegetables, nuts, seeds, and legumes. If you are ordering an entrée, choose an item that is grilled, baked, steamed, or poached instead of fried or sautéed. Also, opt for low-fat dressings and dairy-free options such as olive oil or avocado. Rather than adding a side of French fries or fried onion rings, pick something like roasted sweet potato wedges or a side salad.

If you would like a glass of wine or beer with your meal, several low-alcohol and low-sugar options are available. For dessert, try an item made with fresh fruit such as a parfait or grilled pineapple. Fresh fruit is high in fiber and can help to keep your digestive system running smoothly and free from symptoms.

The key to dining out with diverticulitis is preparation. Take the time to look at the menu beforehand and make a plan so that you can make smart choices. With a little bit of extra effort, you can still enjoy the pleasure of a delicious meal out with your friends and family while following your diverticulitis diet.

Conclusion

Embarking on Your Delicious Healing Journey

You have now worked through the information presented in this cookbook and are equipped with a variety of recipes and tools to assist you in your pursuit of better health through the Diverticulitis Diet. You have been given an overview of which foods to avoid and why, as well as plenty of recipes that are low in fiber and spice but high in flavor. Now is the time to take all of this knowledge and begin creating nutritious and delicious meals to fit within the Diverticulitis Diet guidelines.

Now that you have explored different types of recipes and become familiar with the diet for Diverticulitis, you can use the knowledge to help create your healthy meals. Experiment with different ingredients and seasonings to see what types of flavors you like while still staying within the guidelines of this beneficial diet.

Your journey of good health begins with this cookbook as your guide, but it is up to you to ensure that all of the recipes, food combos, and lifestyle changes you make further promote your journey toward improved wellness.

Once again, job well done on taking the first important step toward taking control of your health by following the Diverticulitis Diet and exploring all the delicious possibilities it contains

Nourishing Your Body, One Meal at a Time

Congratulations on completing your journey to Nourishing Your Body, One Meal at a Time! As you have read, proper nutrition is essential to maintain a healthy body and can positively impact the symptoms of diverticulitis. Eating nutrient-rich meals and a diet low in saturated fat and refined carbohydrates can help you maintain and cultivate a healthy inner ecology and a vibrant relationship with your body.

The recipes and meal plans included in this cookbook provide a variety of options to satisfy your taste buds while still adhering to the diverticulitis diet and lifestyle. We hope these recipes have inspired you to turn healthy ingredients into delicious, nourishing meals.

Remember that the goal of any healthful diet is to always be kind to your body – not just for diverticulitis, but also for overall health and well-being. Eating nutritious meals as outlined in this cookbook is a great way to do just that.

Thank you again for joining us on this journey to cultivating a healthy body and lifestyle for yourself. We wish you the best of luck on your continued journey to health and wellness!